Cinnamon

15 Health Benefits of Cinnamon for Disease Cure, Prevention and Wellness

MARY CONRAD

ISBN: 1532947380
ISBN-13: **978-1532947384**

DEDICATION

This book is for my daughter, Valia, and my supportive husband Vincent. I wouldn't be inspired to write if it wasn't for both of you!

MARY CONRAD

Disclaimer

This book provides general information, personal experiences and extensive research regarding health and related subjects. The information provided in this book, and in any linked materials, is based on my own personal experience and is for informational purposes only. It is not intended to be interpreted as a professional medical advice. Speak with your physician or a trusted healthcare professional prior to taking any nutritional or herbal supplements. Please keep in mind that reactions and results may vary from each individual due to differences in state of health

Before considering any guidance from this book, please ensure you do not have any underlying health conditions, which may interfere with the suggested healing methods. If the reader or any other person has a medical concern or pre-existing condition, please consult with an appropriately licensed physician or healthcare professional. Never disregard professional medical advice or delay in seeking it because of something you have read in this book or in any linked materials.

CONTENTS

INTRODUCTION

Cinnamon is one of my most favorite condiments. Every time I taste that first forkful of apple pie, I sigh at the mix of apple and cinnamon. From the distinct taste to the relaxing aroma, cinnamon is the best spice that brings health benefits and sentimental thoughts.

Cinnamon has been around since the Biblical times, around 2000 B.C. It was used widely in ancient Egypt, as a perfume during the embalming of the dead. In England, it was widely used as a preservative for meat and a status symbol for the wealthy. Today, it is used as a condiment for baking, cooking and added to health drinks all over the world.

Is cinnamon really healthy? The reason why I wrote this book was to share with all of you the great benefits of cinnamon for both health and wellness. The information contained in this eBook is backed up by scientific research or clinical trials. Take the journey with me in discovering the science behind one of the healthiest spice around!

.

Chapter 1

History of Cinnamon

Cinnamon is believed to have been around since 2000 B.C., making it one of the oldest spices used in written history. It's use dates back to ancient Egypt, and was an essential component in the process of embalming. During those times, the popularity of cinnamon was well established, and traders thrived.

The spread of cinnamon to Europe in the Middle Ages was credited to Arab traders, who travelled extensively through difficult land routes. Cinnamon slowly gained a reputation as a status symbol for rich households, who used the spice to preserve meat during the winter months. The increase in demand and limited supply made it even more appealing to the high class society.

The Arab traders refused to reveal where they procured their stocks, and managed to maintain the monopoly and exorbitant price. To dissuade other traders and explorers from ferreting their source of supply, the Arabs spread stories of impossible feats in obtaining the cinnamon sticks. One story claimed that the prized cinnamon sticks were brought to a nest by giant birds. The people who lived near it were said to leave ox meat below the nest, and once the birds took the meat to their nest. The extreme weight topples it over and the people would then collect the sticks.

Despite these rumors, explorers still sought to find the source of the sticks to meet demands. At 1518, it was the Portuguese traders who found the exact location which was in Sri Lanka. There was a power struggle for control of the precious spice between the Portuguese and the Dutch, throwing Sri Lanka in turmoil for almost three centuries. By the 1800, cinnamon had lost its status due to mass cultivation in other parts of the world.

PLANT

Cinnamon belongs to the Cinnamomum genus under the Lauraceae family.

The cinnamon tree is a type of evergreen, which has a soft bark and somewhat small to medium height between 10 to 15 feet. There are two types of cinnamon that are commonly used, which are the Ceylon cinnamon and the cassia cinnamon.

WHAT ARE THE DIFFERENCE BETWEEN THE TWO?

Ceylon Cinnamon

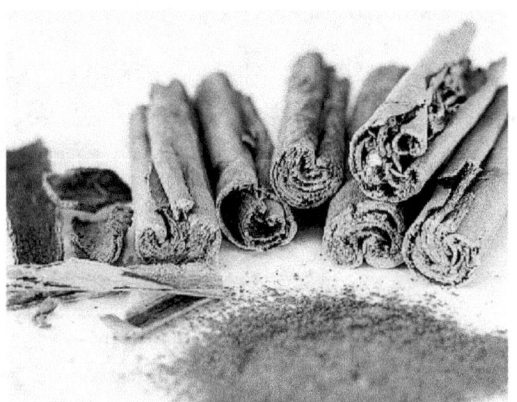

Other names include: Cinnamomum zeylanicum, True Cinnamon, Cinnamomum verum

Ceylon cinnamon is aptly named for its origins. "Ceylon" used to be the name of Sri Lanka around the time when cinnamon was a highly-prized spice. It is predominantly planted and harvested in Sri Lanka, which takes about 80-90% of the worldwide supply for Ceylon cinnamon. The other suppliers include Madagascar, Seychelles and Southern India.

The C. verum cinnamon tree is planted and left to grow and mature for two years. After which, the farmers prune the tree until it appears more like a large shrub.

Right after the rainy season, farmers will begin to harvest the bark. They begin by cutting the small shoots. They wrap it and let it ferment for a certain period of time. It is then stripped of the outer bark. The soft inner bark is removed and stacked. Once it dries, it curls up into "quills" or what is commonly known as cinnamon sticks. The bark near the base of the tree is used for ground cinnamon since it is usually more flavorful.

When purchasing Ceylon cinnamon sticks, you can expect it to be curled, and stuffed on the inside. The taste is mildly sweet and aromatic. It's also low on Coumarin, a bit crumbly with light brown color.

Cassia Cinnamon

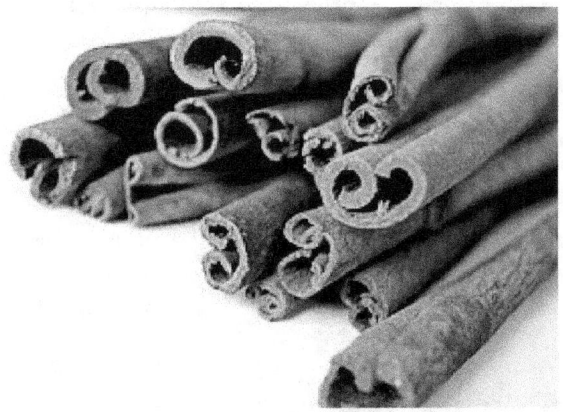

Cassia cinnamon is from other types of cinnamon plants entirely. Those that are classified under "cassia" are Cinnamomum cassia, Cinnamomum burmannii, Cinnamomum loureiroi, and Cinnamomum aromaticum. They are found in Indonesia, Vietnam and China, which supplies the vast majority of cinnamon throughout the world.

Cassia is the predominant type of cinnamon supplied in the United States, with around 20,000-25,000 tons supplied yearly.

The trees are usually left to grow until around ten to fifteen feet. After which, the branches are pruned and the entire bark is stripped off. The bark is then sent to processing in order to remove the outer bark. The inner bark curls right after processing to produce "quills". The sticks produced are often thicker and has a hollow center. This is the visible difference between the two. The lower bark is used for ground cinnamon.

The taste of cassia is a bit spicy and bitter, but with the same aroma as Ceylon. The stick has a darker and richer brown color and thick. Cassia cinnamon has high levels of Coumarin, which can lead to liver failure when taken in excess.

In Europe, Ceylon cinnamon is the almost exclusively used for health and safety purposes. They also require proper labelling, which is not practiced in the United States. Although Ceylon cinnamon is a bit more expensive than cassia, the benefits far outweigh the cost.

AVAILABLE FORMS

There are four available forms of cinnamon, which are ground, sticks, oil extract and capsules/pills.

Ground cinnamon

In the US, ground cinnamon is rarely labelled as Ceylon or cassia. Since cassia is more affordable and easily processed, it makes up the majority of the cinnamon market. This is regardless of the possible health implications of using the spice that has high levels of Coumarin.

If you ever need to use ground cinnamon for baking, cooking or consumption, then make sure to check the source of the cinnamon or for any information that can distinguish it from cassia. In instances where you can't find ground Ceylon cinnamon, you can just buy the sticks and crush it into fine powder by using a mortar or food processor.

Cinnamon sticks

All cinnamon sticks appear as "quills", but the difference between Ceylon and cassia is easy to determine. While cassia sticks are hollow, Ceylon sticks are often stuffed, and appears similar to a cigar.

The taste of Ceylon is mildly sweet, which makes it a great addition to beverages and sweet treats. Cassia has a stronger flavor and spicier.

Cinnamon oil

High quality cinnamon oil is derived from C. verum or C. zeylanicum. The oil is extracted from the leaves and twigs through steam distillation. The parts usually used are those that are left over from pruning. The leaves and twigs are left to dry for a few days prior to the distillation process. Oil derived from the leaves are classified as cinnamon leaf oil, and those that are taken from the bark is labelled as cinnamon bark oil.

Cinnamon oil is listed under GRAS (Generally Recognized As Safe). Some properties of cinnamon oil include:

- antiseptic
- antifungal
- anthelmintic
- anti-diarrheal
- antimicrobial
- antispasmodic
- anti-putrescent
- carminative
- hemostatic

Precautions for Cinnamon oil

1. Cinnamon oil is classified as a "hot" oil, which means it's not a type of oil you can sniff from a bottle. If you want to enjoy it, you would need a diffuser.
2. Some chemical components can cause skin and mucus membrane irritation. When adding this oil in baths, only use half a drop to avoid possible side effects.
3. Avoid ingesting the oil when pregnant or nursing.
4. Keep this oil away from places where kids can find or reach.

For those who want to add cinnamon oil to food or beverage, choose cinnamon bark oil. The oil derived exclusively from the bark is easier to digest and more refined. Consult a professional before using the oil in order to determine the dosage and monitor safety.

Cinnamon Tablets

There are cinnamon supplements available in tablet form. These would be a great help when you want to get the benefits without having to brew a cup of tea. A few reminders when using tablets:
- Check the purity of the cinnamon used. There may be fillers or chemicals added to avoid clumping or preserve the quality of cinnamon.
- Always check with your naturopathic doctor before using this to avoid possible complications.

STORAGE

To fully enjoy the flavor of cinnamon, choose the organically grown variety. This will ensure maximum flavor minus the possible side effects of irradiation. Store the ground cinnamon or cinnamon sticks in a glass airtight container. Place it away from direct heat, sunlight and moisture. You can extend shelf life by keeping it in the refrigerator.

Ground cinnamon can be stored for up to six months. Cinnamon sticks can last up to a year with proper storage. You can determine whether it is fresh or not by smelling it. If it still has a sweet smell then it's still good to use, if not then it should be discarded.

WHAT TO EXPECT WHEN TAKING CINNAMON

1. There are usually no side effects of using cinnamon, but excessive consumption may cause irritation on the lips and mouth. Some experience skin irritation and slight inflammation when taking it in large quantities.

2. Cassia cinnamon is not meant to be consumed at high quantities. It has considerable levels of Coumarin which can lead to liver failure, especially for those who have predisposed conditions.

3. Those with diabetes need to be cautious when taking cinnamon for supplements. It enhances the effect of insulin, so there may be a need to adjust the insulin dosage.

4. There are no general guidelines for taking cinnamon, so for those who are pregnant, nursing and children below six years old should not take cinnamon supplements. Better safe than sorry!

5. Before taking cinnamon supplements, consult your healthcare professional. It could be your holistic doctors, herbalist or naturopathic physicians. This is a must, especially for those who are taking antibiotics, blood thinners or any maintenance medication.

NUTRITIONAL PROFILE

Ground cinnamon: 2 tsp (5.20 g)

BASIC MACRONUTRIENTS AND CALORIES
Nutrient: Amount
Protein:0.21 g
Carbohydrate:4.19 g
Fat total: 0.06 g
Dietary Fiber:2.76 g
Calories: 12.84

MACRONUTRIENT AND CALORIE DETAIL
Nutrient: Amount
Carbohydrate:
Total Sugars: 0.11 g
Monosaccharides: 0.11 g
Fructose:0.06 g
Glucose:0.05 g
Other Carbohydrates:1.32 g

Fat:
Monounsaturated Fat:0.01 g
Saturated Fat:0.02 g
Calories from Fat:0.58
Calories from Sat. Fat:0.16
Water :0.55 g

MICRONUTRIENTS
Nutrient: Amount
Vitamins:
Water-Soluble Vitamins
B-Complex Vitamins
Vitamin B3: 0.07 mg
Vitamin B3:0.11 mg
Vitamin B6: 0.01 mg
Choline:0.57 mg
Folate: 0.31 mcg
Folate (DFE):0.31 mcg
Folate (food) :0.31 mcg
Pantothenic Acid:0.02 mg
Vitamin C:0.20 mg

Fat-Soluble Vitamins
Vitamin A (Retinoids and Carotenoids)
Vitamin A International Units (IU) :15.34 IU
Alpha-Carotene: 0.05 mcg
Beta-Carotene: 5.82 mcg
Beta-Carotene Equivalents:9.20 mcg
Cryptoxanthin:6.71 mcg
Lutein and Zeaxanthin:11.54 mcg
Lycopene:0.78 mcg

Vitamin E
Vitamin E International Units (IU) :0.18 IU
Vitamin E mg: 0.12 mg
Vitamin K:1.62 mcg

Minerals:
Nutrient: Amount
Calcium:52.10 mg
Copper:0.02 mg
Iron :0.43 mg
Magnesium:3.12 mg
Manganese:0.91 mg
Phosphorus:3.33 mg
Potassium:22.41 mg
Selenium: 0.16 mcg
Sodium:0.52 mg
Zinc :0.10 mg

INDIVIDUAL FATTY ACIDS
Nutrient: Amount
18:1 Oleic:0.01 g

POLYUNSATURATED FATTY ACIDS
Nutrient: Amount
16:0 Palmitic:0.01 g
17:0 Margaric:0.01 g

INDIVIDUAL AMINO ACIDS
Nutrient: Amount
Alanine: 0.01 g
Arginine: 0.01 g
Aspartic Acid:0.02 g

Glutamic Acid: 0.02 g
Glycine: 0.01 g
Histidine: 0.01 g
Isoleucine: 0.01 g
Leucine: 0.01 g
Lysine:0.01 g
Phenylalanine: 0.01 g
Proline: 0.02 g
Serine: 0.01 g
Threonine: 0.01 g
Tyrosine: 0.01 g
Valine: 0.01 g

Chapter 2

Healthy Cinnamon Recipes

1. Cinnamon Black Tea Infusion
This infusion is a great way to start your morning.

Ingredients:
- o   2 Ceylon Cinnamon sticks/ 1 tsp Ground Ceylon Cinnamon
- o   3 cups of water
- o   1 black tea bags (Ceylon, Nepali or your own personal preference)
- o   sugar cubes (optional substitute: maple syrup or honey)

How to make:

1.   In a saucepan, add three cups of water. Add the cinnamon sticks and let it boil for 15 minutes. It takes about 15 minutes for the sticks to release their flavor into the water.

For ground cinnamon, you can determine whether it's done by the color. It will turn the mixture into a deep brown color.

2. Transfer into a pot and add the black tea bags. Let it steep for a 2-3 minutes. You can also use loose tea if you prefer.
3. Add sugar cubes for sweetness. Serve.

2. Cinnamon-Ginger Cold Cure

Ingredients:

- o   1/4 cup of sliced or crushed ginger
- o   1 tsp ground cinnamon
- o   2 cups water
- o   2 lemons (juice both)
- o   2 tbsp. raw honey

How to make:

1. In a pot, add water, ginger and cinnamon. Boil for 15 minutes.
2. In two separate cups, divide the lemon juice and add one tbsp. of honey each. Stir until the honey is incorporated into the juice.
3. Strain the ginger-cinnamon mixture into the cups. Let it cool and serve.

3. Soothing Lemon Cinnamon Tea

Ingredients:
- o   4 cups of water
- o   2 Cinnamon sticks
- o   2 cloves
- o   2 bags of your preferred tea
- o   4 tbsp. lemon juice
- o   2 tbsp. of brown sugar

How to make:

1. In a pot, add water, cloves and cinnamon. Let it boil for 10-15 minutes.
2. Remove from heat and add the tea bags. Let it steep for 3-5 minutes.
3. Discard the bags, and add the lemon juice at small intervals. Make sure you taste it to ensure that it's to your liking.
4. Warm the mixture under low heat. Strain the mixture into your cup. Add sugar or any sweetener of your preference.

4. *Warm Spiced Persimmon Tea*

Ingredients:

- o   8 cups
- o   2 inches fresh, sliced & mildly crushed ginger
- o   2 inches sliced turmeric root
- o   1 tsp of fresh peppercorns
- o   6 Ceylon Cinnamon sticks
- o   1 large fuyu persimmon, sliced thinly
- o   Stevia/Honey/Sugar

How to make:

1. In a large saucepan, add all the ingredients. Let it simmer under low heat for 20-30 minutes.
2. Strain the mixture into a container.
3. Pour into cups, and sweeten as per preference.

5. Carrot-Cinnamon Smoothie

Ingredients:
- o 2 medium-sized carrots (choose organic if possible)
- o 1 fresh mango, sliced into chunks
- o 50 grams of frozen pineapple chunks
- o 1/2 banana
- o 1 tbsp. flax seeds
- o 1/4 tsp ground Ceylon Cinnamon
- o 2 cups water
- o 1/4 cup strawberries

Instructions:

1. Clean the carrots and chop off both ends. Slice into smaller pieces, and toss it in a blender. Add all the other ingredients.
2. Blend it until smooth. Serve.

6. Delicious Mexican Horchata

Ingredients
- o   1 ⅔ cups uncooked white long-grain rice
- o   5 cups water
- o   2 Ceylon cinnamon sticks
- o   ½ cup white sugar
- o   3 cups milk
- o   2 tsp. vanilla
- o   Ice cubes

How to make:

1. In a blender, pour two cups of water and rice. Blend for one minute. Pour three more cups of water, and blend for 30 seconds.
2. Set aside the mixture for at least three hours. Strain the mixture, and discard the rice. Add the rest of the ingredients and stir until well incorporated.
3. Let it chill for a few hours. Pour into ice-filled glass and enjoy!

7. *Vegan Strawberry Shortcake Smoothie*

Ingredients:

- o 3 cups frozen strawberries
- o 1¾ cup nondairy milk of your choice
- o ¼ cup cashew butter
- o 5 dates
- o 1 tsp pure vanilla extract
- o 1 tsp cinnamon
- o ⅓ cup oats (not the instant variety)

How to make:

1. Throw it all in the blender. Pulse and blend until smooth. The consistency is thick so it may take a while to blend it well.

8. Apple Cinnamon Infused Water

Ingredients:
- o   2 Ceylon cinnamon sticks
- o   1 liter of water
- o   2 lemons

How to make:

1. Prepare a large pitcher with a wide opening. Slice both apples into thin strips, and place it in the pitcher. Add the two sticks of cinnamon. Squeeze the lemon juice and pour the water.
2. Set aside the mixture for one day. Drink up and enjoy!

Note: You can top it up with up to three liters of water.

9. *Chai and Cinnamon Latte*

Ingredients
- o   1 Chai Spice black tea bag
- o   1/4 cup hot water
- o   3/4 cup Whole Milk
- o   Honey or Stevia
- o   Cinnamon, Cardamom, and Nutmeg to taste

How to make:

1.   Steep the Chai tea bag in hot water for 5 minutes.
2.   In a saucepan, warm the milk while whisking. Remove from heat. Pour the Chai tea, and stir to combine. Add milk and honey to taste.
3.   Add a dash of cinnamon, nutmeg and cardamom. Serve.

10. Hearty Oatmeal Shake

Ingredients:
- o   1/2 cup gluten-free instant oats
- o   2 cups water
- o   1 cup fat free milk (or any milk of your choice)
- o   1 cup ice
- o   3 tbsp. sugar
- o   2 tsp ground cinnamon

How to make:

1. In a small pot, cook the oats. Mix often until it becomes thick. Set aside to cool.
2. In a blender, pour in the milk. Add the cinnamon, sugar, oats and ice. Turn the blender on high and mix until smooth.

Chapter 3

Cinnamon and Diabetes

Diabetes mellitus is a chronic health condition that requires lifelong management. It's a state where there is a significant and consistent elevation in a person's blood sugar levels. This occurs due to: low levels of insulin in the body, the lack of cells which produce insulin or inability of the body to respond to insulin.

The hormone insulin is produced in the pancreas by beta-cells. Their main function is to assist in the uptake of glucose by the cells. It allows the large glucose molecule to pass into the cell to be used for energy or stored for later use.

There are two types of diabetes: Type 1 (Insulin-Dependent) and Type 2 (Non-insulin Dependent).

Type 1 Diabetes Mellitus

Type 1 Diabetes is a condition wherein the immune system fights off the cells that produce insulin leaving insufficient amounts of the hormone in the body.

This type is actually not common. Only 10% of those diagnosed with Diabetes are under this classification, and are usually determined by the age of 40.

Causes:

The main cause of this type of diabetes is still unknown. It's basically an autoimmune disorder that has a slow onset as the immune system gradually destroys the beta-cells in the pancreas.

There are a few possible reasons that could explain the cause:

1. Genes: About 90% of those who have Type 1 DM have a history of the condition within the family. There may be susceptible genes that trigger the immune system to attack the cells in the pancreas. Ethnic groups such as Scandinavian and Sardinians are also more likely to develop the condition.

2. Autoantigen: This protein is released when there is injury to the pancreas such as during infections. It is believed to trigger the T-cell-mediated immune response thereby destroying beta cells. But it looks to be a response to the injury and not the direct cause of β-cell death.

3. Viruses: There are a few viruses that trigger the autoimmune response by damaging the β-cells or cause autoantigens to be released; this leads to an autoreactive immune response. The viruses include: coxsackievirus, rubella virus, cytomegalovirus, Epstein-Barr virus, and retroviruses.

4. Diet: According to findings, infants who are fed cow's milk, milk protein β casein, high nitrates in drinking water, and vitamin D deficits have increased chances of developing type 1 DM. Early consumption of gluten and cereals, between 4-7 months also increases autoantibody productions.

Type 2 Diabetes Mellitus

Type 2 Diabetes is a condition wherein the body has developed a resistance to insulin, which makes the circulating levels inadequate. It's either the liver is constantly producing glucose or the cells in the body can no longer detect insulin.

One of the major causes for developing this type of diabetes is obesity. Research has found that obesity is a stressor for individual cells. The persistent high levels of glucose, either through intake or lipolysis, causes the cell to react. Once there is too much nutrients (glucose) inside the cell, the endoplasmic reticulum sends out an alarm to the membrane to reduce the insulin receptors on the cell wall, which stops the glucose from entering. This in turn allows the cell to use up the nutrients and maintain balance. Eventually, persistent high glucose intake will continue to overwork the cells and it would continue the cycle to the point of insulin resistance.

HOW CINNAMON AFFECT BLOOD SUGAR LEVELS

Cinnamon extracts show to have significant effects on blood sugar levels by increasing insulin sensitivity in the cells. According to a recent study, it has the ability to prevent the development of insulin resistance, partly by increasing the insulin sensitivity through the nitric oxide pathways found in the skeletal muscles. Aqueous extracts also show the same effect.

In the blood stream, cinnamon extracts also assist in facilitating the entry of glucose into the cell. It affects glucose-uptake related genes such as Glut1, Glut4, glycogen synthesis 1, and glycogen synthase kinase 3β mRNA expression in adipose tissue. This allows for the transport of glucose molecules into the cell, which in effect lowers the serum glucose levels.

HOW TO TAKE CINNAMON FOR DIABETES

Cinnamon is only effective for Type 2 DM. Some studies suggest that cassia cinnamon may be more effective for diabetes, but they actually have similar therapeutic effects. For safety purposes, it would be preferable to use Ceylon Cinnamon due to its reduced levels of Coumarin. With the potential complications of having DM, it would be much better to use a safer but effective option.

To take cinnamon powder for diabetes, the advised dosage is about 1.25 teaspoon once daily for five days, with two days of rest. This is to avoid toxicity or build up.

For cinnamon sticks, it would be best to create tea in order to get the maximum effect. You can create cinnamon stick tea by boiling two cups of water. Add two Ceylon cinnamon sticks, and boil it for 15 minutes until the color of the water turns light brown. You can drink this straight or add a sweetener such as stevia or honey.

Cinnamon bark oil is one of the more effective forms in lowering blood glucose levels. Due to its higher concentration, it only takes about 1-2 drops of the oil mixed with food or beverage to get the desired effect. Before using this form, it would be best to consult your naturopathic or holistic health professionals. The main reason is because of the risk for hypoglycemia, especially at concentrated doses, as well as possible stomach irritation.

Chapter 4

Cinnamon and Yeast Infection

Yeast infection is a condition that occurs when fungi, such as Candida, multiply at a rapid rate causing discomfort. The skin's surface as well as the mucosa is home to other microorganisms. During cases wherein there is an imbalance in the body, these organisms start taking over the area by reproducing at an accelerated rate. This imbalance may be due to taking antibiotics or when the person's immune system is suppressed.

This infection is commonly caused by Candida albicans, which is present in the skin and mucosa. It can occur in different areas such as the mouth, esophagus, vagina, skin and the blood stream (rare but possibly fatal).

Common Causes of Yeast Infection

- Use of antibiotics - kills off lactobacillus that help maintain pH in the vagina, which results in the overgrowth of the fungi.
- Pregnancy

- Hormone therapy/oral contraceptives
- Those with low immunity
- Untreated diabetes
- Stress

Signs and Symptoms

The primary signs and symptoms of candidiasis are:
- White, curd-like discharge from the vagina/white lesions on the oral cavity
- Redness, soreness on the affected area
- Itchiness or general discomfort such as burning and pain during intercourse

HOW CINNAMON AFFECTS YEAST INFECTION

Recent studies have supported the effectiveness of cinnamon as an antifungal. In the Journal of Traditional Medicine, a study used cinnamon oil mixed with pogostemon oil to observe how Candida albicans, Candida tropicalis, and Candida krusei, react to this treatment.

The experiment utilized a mixture of the oils at different concentrations for each strain. The observed effect of the treatment in vitro was a rapid destruction of the fungi cells. The organelles of the cells hollowed out, killing it from the inside. Within 48-72 hours, all that was left of the cells were empty cytoplasms. They also conducted the study on a group of 60 people who had intestinal candidiasis. These individuals were given capsules of the same mixture of cinnamon oil and pogostemon oil. The results marked a significant antifungal effect of both oils in all strains of Candida.

HOW TO TAKE CINNAMON FOR YEAST INFECTION

Taking cinnamon for yeast infection can be done safely.

Cinnamon Tea (Ceylon Cinnamon): You can use the recipe for Cinnamon Black Tea Infusion as a daily regimen to prevent recurrence of infection. Black tea contains polyphenols that also adds an antifungal effect to the beverage, which makes it a great addition to your morning routine. Just remember to have rest days each week to avoid toxicity.

Another way of taking cinnamon minus the black tea, is by boiling about two cups of water and two Ceylon cinnamon sticks (1 and 1/2 tsp of ground cinnamon) for about 15 minutes or until the water turns light to deep brown. Ceylon cinnamon is naturally sweet so there's no need to add any sweetener.

Before considering taking cinnamon bark oil or cinnamon leaf oil internally, always consult a professional in order to mix the correct dosages and concentrations. These two oils are concentrated and need careful handling.

Topical use of cinnamon leaf oil is possible for skin candidiasis. You can create a mixture by adding 1% of cinnamon leaf oil to a carrier oil such as almond oil, apricot oil or olive oil. Make sure to avoid any possible contact with genitals, mouth and eyes.

To make the treatment more effective, go on a Candida diet and avoid sweets, yeasty breads or pastries. Sadly, chocolates are also part of the list to avoid.

PRECAUTIONS

It's always best to go to a physician for a diagnosis if you suspect that you have candidiasis, especially if this is the first time you've acquired the infection, pregnant or have a 101 °F fever and lower abdominal pain.

MARY CONRAD

Chapter 5

Cinnamon and Stomach Flu

Stomach flu or gastroenteritis is an infection that is manifested by diarrhea, vomiting, nausea, abdominal pain and fever. This condition is marked by inflammation of the gastrointestinal tract from bacteria or viruses.

The infection is commonly acquired through contaminated water or food.

COMMON CAUSES OF STOMACH FLU

Virus:

1. Rotavirus: This is the most common cause of stomach flu for children. It usually takes a period of two days before the symptoms appear. It can last 3-8 days with marked vomiting and

diarrhea.

2. <u>Norovirus</u>: This is a contagious virus that is the most common cause of food poisoning. It can cause stomach pain, vomiting and diarrhea. It can be passed through contaminated food and water, as well as contact with a contaminated person. It usually takes 12-48 hours to manifest symptoms, and 1-3 days to clear up on its own.

Bacteria:

1. <u>Yersinia</u>: Is a common infection for children, which is marked by fever, abdominal pain and bloody diarrhea. Symptoms are often manifested between 4-7 days after exposure. It can last between 1-3 weeks, and may require medical attention. It is usually found in pork meat, specifically near the tonsils.

2. <u>Staphylococcus</u>: This infection has an onset of about 2 days after ingestion of contaminated food. It takes about 3 days to clear out on its own. The severity depends on the current health status. It is usually found in dairy products, meat, and eggs.

3. <u>Shigella</u>: Is another common infection for toddlers during the summer months. It is associated with water contaminated with feces, as well as contaminated food. The symptoms often manifest after a day of exposure. It takes around 5-7 days for the infection to clear out.

4. <u>Salmonella</u>: This bacterium is often found in beef, dairy and eggs. It's often a result of poor food handling. The symptoms may develop after 12-72 hours, and take 4-7 days to leave the system. It may be several months before bowel movement will return to normal. A few of those infected may develop Reiter's syndrome, which can last for years and eventually lead to arthritis.

5. <u>Campylobacter</u>: This is a common cause of infection in the UK. It's usually found in undercooked meat, especially poultry. It takes about 2-5 days for symptoms to show, and about a week to pass out of the body.

6. <u>E. coli</u>: This is often the reason behind food poisoning for travelers. It takes about 24-72 hours before symptoms can be experienced. A strain of this bacteria (E. coli O157:H7) can

cause severe food poisoning.

HOW CINNAMON AFFECTS STOMACH FLU

In vitro and in vivo studies have proven that cinnamon may be effective in destroying E. coli, Staphylococcus, Salmonella and Campylobacter. These studies utilized Cinnamon zeylanicum extracts in determining the antibacterial properties of cinnamon. The results showed that there is a significant inhibition of the spread of the bacteria listed above. Although further human testing needs to be done to note bioavailability and absorption rates.

Antiviral properties of cinnamon have been studied as well. Cinnamon oil from C. zeylanicum has shown to inhibit the growth of human rotavirus.

HOW TO TAKE CINNAMON FOR STOMACH FLU

The great thing about cinnamon is that you don't need it to be in a capsule. It's actually quite good as a tea or beverage.

Cinnamon stick tea: Choose the Ceylon cinnamon stick variety when making this tea. It not only tastes better, it's also safer to drink. Boil about two cups of water. Add the Ceylon cinnamon sticks, and let it boil for 15 minutes. Once the water turns light to deep brown, you can remove it from the heat. Let it cool and transfer into a cup and drink. You can add a sweetener if preferred but it's usually not needed. Ceylon cinnamon sticks are often mildly sweet.

Ground Cinnamon: It's always best to choose a good quality cinnamon, preferably the Ceylon variety. Boil about two cups of water. Add one and a half teaspoon of cinnamon powder. Let it simmer for at 15 minutes. Strain then set aside to cool, add a teaspoon of honey. Serve.

You can also opt to add ginger while boiling to add to the antibacterial effect. Ginger also helps with inflammation and nausea. If there are issues with dehydration, you can add 1/4 teaspoon of salt and 1 teaspoon of sugar. This can assist with rehydration. Keep in mind that small sips are more effective than gulping it all down. Sudden oral rehydration will only upset the stomach and induce either vomiting or diarrhea.

PRECAUTIONS:

There are warning signs you should always keep in mind when it comes to stomach flu. Excessive vomiting and diarrhea can lead to dehydration. Take note of the signs of severe dehydration, such as:

- Sunken fontanels in infants
- Sleepiness in children and infants
- Sunken eyes
- Fever
- Absence of tears when crying
- Dry skin (Do a pinch test. Take a small patch of skin between your fingers. Pull on it slightly. If it takes more than five seconds to return to normal, then it's positive for dehydration)
- Low urine output (If there is any, it's often concentrated and very yellow)
- Extreme thirst
- Low blood pressure
- Heartbeat is fast as well as breathing

If any of the above symptoms are noted, this requires emergency medical assistance. For infants, young children and older adults it's best to have them on Intravenous Infusion once there are signs of dehydration. It might be best to see a health professional if the child is having severe diarrhea and vomiting for over 24 hours, black or bloody stools and trouble drinking.

When taking cinnamon tea, please make sure there are rest days each week to prevent toxicity.

Chapter 6

Cinnamon for Irritable Bowel Syndrome

Irritable Bowel Syndrome (IBS) affects the large intestines. It is often marked by bloating, gas, diarrhea, constipation and abdominal cramps. Although it can be painful and quite uncomfortable, it can be managed through lifestyle and diet.

CAUSES FOR IBS

There is no specific cause of IBS. There seems to be poor signal coordination between the nerves and the muscles of the large intestines which causes it to either not contract properly (constipation) or have excessive motility (diarrhea). There are several possible triggers for this particular condition such as:

- *Food*: Different people have different food triggers. It is always best to determine what food sets the condition off. A food diary is a great way of keeping track. There also commonly reported irritants such as dairy, spices, fats, fruits, alcohol and carbonated drinks.

- *Stress:* This often aggravates the symptoms of IBS.

- *Hormones:* This condition occurs more in females than in males, so it is believed that hormones have some effect on the occurrence of IBS.

- *Overrun of bad bacteria:* When there's an overrun of bad bacteria in the gut, it can trigger IBS. This can be prevented by regular intake of probiotics.

HOW CINNAMON AFFECTS IBS

A study was conducted to observe the effects of natural remedies on symptoms of IBS. The goal was to improve bowel movements and habits. It utilized two different mixtures of natural remedies. One mixture was made with dried, powdered bilberry fruit, slippery elm bark, agrimony aerial parts, and cinnamon quills. The second mixture was made with dried powdered slippery elm bark, lactulose, oat bran, and licorice root. The results revealed that the first and second mixture were both effective in relieving the symptoms of IBS but the second mixture was able to normalize the bowel movements and consistency.

Although the study showed that cinnamon can help with alleviating the symptoms, it might be a possible trigger for IBS as well. So it might be a good idea to try it out first before using it as a treatment. Not everyone reacts to potential triggers, it's always best to note your own reactions.

HOW TO TAKE CINNAMON FOR IBS

Cinnamon helps relieve the symptoms of IBS, such as bloating, gas and abdominal cramps.

Cinnamon Tea: You can use cinnamon tea to alleviate the symptoms as well as rehydrate. Boil two cinnamon stick, preferably the Ceylon variety, in two cups of water. Add 1/4 teaspoon and salt and 1 teaspoon of sugar. Let it boil for 15 minutes. Let it cool, and take sips throughout the day.

For diarrhea, you can make your own homemade rehydrating solution. Take about 240 ml of filtered water. Add 1/4 teaspoon of salt, and 1 teaspoon of water. Stir until everything dissolves. Drink for every episode of diarrhea, just make sure to drink at small increments. This is to maintain osmotic pressure so water will be retained.

PRECAUTIONS

It is best to avoid ingesting high doses of cinnamon powder or even a drop of cinnamon oil when pregnant and nursing. For children, ground cinnamon may be added to food in small amounts.

Before using cinnamon oil for ingestion or therapeutic uses other than diffusion, consult a professional to avoid unnecessary complications.

Chapter 7

Cinnamon for Cancer Prevention

Cancer is an abnormal proliferation of cells. It is marked by mutated cells that reproduce at a fast rate, and clump together forming tumors. There are over 100 types of cancer, each with different methods of diagnosis and treatment.

CAUSES OF CANCER

There are several determined causes of cancer.

- *Genetics:* This factor has been linked primarily as a major cause for cancer. A genetic mutation causes the cell to multiply rapidly, grow uncontrollably and unable to repair the mutation.

  Tumor suppressor genes are the ones responsible in triggering the stop of cell growth and division. If these genes are turned off or not functioning, it would leave the cell to continue growing and multiplying. These cells use up resources at rapid rates, which leaves the healthy cells with little.

DNA repair genes are the ones responsible for correcting any errors or mutations. When this is suppressed, the mutated cells will not be fixed.

These mutations can either be something you're born with or developed due to other factors listed below.

- *Environmental Factors:* Exposure to UV rays, radiation, bacteria and carcinogens increases the risk of developing cancer. Another example is exposure to sunlight during peak hours of 10 A.M. to 3 P.M., when UV rays cause the most damage.

- *Lifestyle:* Some habits have been proven to cause cancer, such as tobacco smoking, passive smoking, excessive use of tanning beds and excessive intake of alcohol.

GENERAL SIGNS AND SYMPTOMS

These are signs and symptoms that are linked to cancer, but are not definitive until further testing.

- Changes in weight, such as excessive loss or gain
- Changes in skin color, such as darkening or yellowing
- Fatigue
- Presence of lumps or irregularities under the skin
- Sores that are not healing
- Changes in existing moles
- Sudden changes in bowel or bladder routines
- Hoarseness
- Chronic discomforts in eating, swallowing and digestion
- Unexplained muscle or joint pain
- On and off fever and night sweats
- Sudden, unexplained bleeding and bruising

HOW CINNAMON PREVENTS CANCER

Several studies have proven the positive effects of cinnamon for certain types of cancer. These were conducted through microscope and animal tests. The results shed a positive light for the use of cinnamon for both treatment and prevention.

Stops tumor growth and spread

In a recent study, cinnamaldehyde, specifically 2'-Hydroxycinnamaldehyde and 2'-benzoyloxycinnamaldehyde, showed to stop the growth of 29 types of human cancer cells in vitro. The results hint at the anticancer properties of cinnamon on the cellular level. Further testing on humans may still be needed to fully explore the potential of cinnamon as treatment.

Induces apoptosis

Cinnamaldehyde induces apoptosis or cell death by increasing the permeability of the cancer cell membrane. The reactive oxygen species is produced which alters the mitochondria leading to apoptosis.

Modulates T-cell differentiation

Isolated 2'-Hydroxycinnamaldehyde and 2'-benzoyloxycinnamaldehyde has shown to inhibit growth of abnormal lymphocytes and trigger T-cell differentiation. This blocks the signaling pathways for abnormal cell growth.

HOW TO TAKE CINNAMON FOR CANCER PREVENTION

There is still a need to test out cinnamon's effectiveness for actual treatment of cancer. For prevention purposes, a regular intake through diet can go a long way in achieving health. Any of the beverage recipes in this book taken regularly with rest days may do wonders in avoiding this dreaded disease.

PRECAUTIONS

Taking cinnamon in dietary dosages is generally considered safe. Those that are pregnant, nursing and children under six years should be cautious in terms of amount consumed. Cassia cinnamon may cause liver problems, ensure that you're healthy prior to making any dietary modifications.

Chapter 8

Cinnamon for Bone Health

The skeletal system is made up of about 206 bones for adults. It is well known that our bones support our body by providing a framework for muscles and tendons, but it has several more functions that are equally as important.

- *Support and Movement*: Joints help increase the range of motion and allow movement.

- *Protection*: The skull, ribs and vertebrae protect major organs from potential trauma.

- *Storage:* Bones store calcium which can be released when there are low levels of calcium in the body. It also stores ferritin, which helps iron storage and metabolism.

- *Blood Cell Production:* The bone marrow is responsible for the production of red and white blood cells. Not all bones produce blood cells, only those located in the pelvis, sternum, vertebrae and cranium.

- *Hormone Release:* Osteocalcin is released by bone cells. It contributes to insulin sensitivity, increased levels and reduction of fat stores.

The bone density reaches its peak at the age of 30. After which, there tends to be natural bone degeneration with age, lifestyle, dietary factors and illnesses.

HOW CINNAMON AFFECTS BONE HEALTH

A study conducted sought to observe the effects of C. zeylanicum on osteoclastogenesis or osteoclast formation. Osteoclasts are the cells responsible for the breakdown of calcium from the bone to the blood stream. There is a delicate balance between calcium storage and calcium breakdown in the body. In certain conditions, such as osteoporosis, bone cancer and metastasis and rheumatoid arthritis, there is an increase in osteoclastogenesis. This increases the breakdown of calcium in the bones, making it more brittle and hollow.

After using C. zeylanicum extracts, there was a marked inhibition of osteoclastogenesis. The two main compounds responsible were cinnamaldehyde and 2-methoxycinnamaldehyde. They act on the nuclear factor of activated T cell 1 (NFATc1) pathway, which plays an active role in osteoclast formation, by inhibiting receptor activation on the cells. It even affects mature osteoclast activity by reducing bone resorption.

Overall, the findings bring a different approach in the treatment of bone diseases as well as prevention of secondary bone degeneration.

There is a potential anti-inflammatory effect of cinnamon as well. According to a study, the extract of C. osmophleum showed a significant anti-inflammatory properties based on the chemical composition of the extract. This effect requires further research for development.

HOW TO TAKE CINNAMON FOR BONE HEALTH

The best method of preserving bone health is through prevention by occasional weight-bearing exercises, range-of-motion exercises and a healthy lifestyle and diet. Adding cinnamon tea and other beverages would be a great start in keeping the bones healthy.

A brand of water-based cinnamon supplement, Cinnulin PF, is derived from Cassia cinnamon. It isolated the therapeutic components of cassia while removing the harmful chemicals. Therapeutic dosages of cinnamon would require further assessment by a professional prior to intake.

PRECAUTIONS

Be vigilant when combining prescription medications with cinnamon. There could be possible interactions. Cinnamon can act as a blood thinner, so for those who will undergo surgery, have bleeding disorders or liver problems; exercise caution when taking this supplement.

Pregnant, nursing mothers and children should only take cinnamon in moderate dietary amounts.

.

Chapter 9

Antimicrobial Properties of Cinnamon

The antimicrobial properties of cinnamon have been discovered long before any studies were conducted. It was used as meat preservative in England during the Middle Ages by rich households. They had use it quite effectively and it was prized for its multiple uses and expensive price.

WHAT ARE THE ACTIVE CHEMICAL COMPONENTS OF CINNAMON?

A study sought to find the antimicrobial properties of 21 essential oils. There were only two essential oils, which includes cinnamon oil, that proved to be effective against both Gram positive and Gram negative bacteria.

By using Gas chromatography mass spectrometry (GC/MS), they broke down the major chemical components of cinnamon. After identifying 38 phytochemicals, they determined the major components, which are: cinnamaldehyde, benzaldehyde, benzoic acid and benzyl alcohol. Cinnamaldehyde comprised the majority of the compounds in the extracts.

ANTIBACTERIAL ACTION

The hydrophobic properties of the essential oils allow it to break into the lipids of the bacteria's cell membrane and mitochondria. This makes it more permeable, with ions and nutrients passing out of the cell uncontrollably, which causes the cell to eventually die.

HOW TO TAKE CINNAMON FOR ANTIMICROBIAL BENEFITS

Cinnamon oil needs to be diluted when taken internally. To increase immunity and gut health, you can place one to two drops of oil in an empty vegetable capsule.

Cinnamon tea is also a great way to get its benefits. The oil can also be added to your favorite tea. One drop of cinnamon oil in your tea can help with stomach flu and throat infections.

PRECAUTIONS

Small doses of cinnamon oil are considered safe and effective in inhibiting bacteria growth. With the help of an herbalist, it can be added to beverage, but be reminded that it needs to be heavily diluted. The same principle is true for topical application; it would need to be mixed with carrier oils.

It can't be given internally for pregnant or nursing mothers. Topical application is also not advised. For children over 6 years old, it can be used topically and internally with heavy dilution. Consult your naturopathic doctor or herbalist to determine the right dose per weight, especially for children.

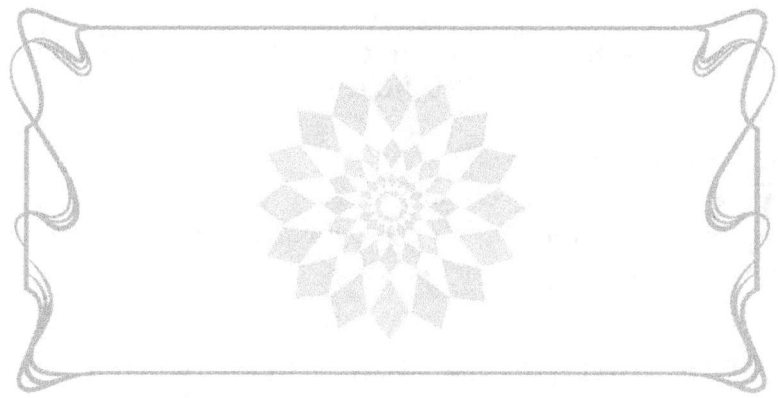

Chapter 10

Improved Alertness and Cognitive Function

Despite the wide array of modern technology at our disposal, the mind still continues to amaze us with its versatility. There is still so much of our brain that remains a mystery. The limits of what our brain can learn and relearn is not fully known.

Cognitive function involves any activity that leads to learning. This includes memory, comprehension, reasoning, language and attention. It is often affected by external and internal factors, such as physical health, emotions and environmental conditions.

COMMON COGNITIVE FUNCTION DISORDERS INCLUDE:

- Dementia
- Amnesia
- Developmental Disorders

- Motor skills disorders

COMMON CAUSES FOR COGNITIVE FUNCTION DISORDERS

- Physical trauma
- Hormonal imbalances during life in the womb
- Lack of essential nutrients during cognitive developmental stages
- Substance abuse (alcohol and drugs)

DOES COGNITIVE FUNCTION DECLINE WITH AGE?

According to Emory University's Alzheimer's Disease Research Center, there are several misconceptions about the decline of cognition with aging.

Although aging does slow down the conversion of recent memories to long term memory, remote memories are often sharp and retained. Knowledge derived from experience also remain intact, whereas those that are not, may decline. Focused attention, or paying attention to one aspect is still maintained through aging, but those activities which require attention to be divided becomes challenging. Language and vocabulary prove to remain constant as we age, but retrieval of words and details during conversation will be more difficult. The speed of data processing also takes more time as aging affects the cognitive and motor processes.

There is a natural form of decline, but despite that there are ways of keeping the brain sharp and active. Activities such as reading, learning new skills, exercising memory, comprehension and other functions will keep the brain in better condition as we age. A healthy diet and lifestyle also play a role in keeping the brain active.

HOW CINNAMON AFFECTS ALERTNESS AND COGNITIVE FUNCTION

A study from the Wheeling Jesuit University, sought to determine the relationship between the odor (orthonasal vs. retronasal) and cognitive function. The subjects were divided for two different phases of the study.

Phase 1 sought to study the effects of retronasal odors by having the subjects eat chewing gum while completing tasks on a program that measures levels of cognition. Thirty-one volunteers were divided into five groups: unflavored, cinnamon gum, peppermint gum, cherry gum and the control group.

Phase 2 studied the effects of orthonasal odors and cognitive function by having the respondents finish tasks with a nasal cannula containing low flow oxygen mixed with three different oils. Thirty-nine subjects were divided into four groups: cinnamon, peppermint, jasmine and the control group.

The results for both showed marked increase in cognitive function for those who had used both the cinnamon flavored gum and diffused cinnamon oil. The cognitive tasks included attentional processes, virtual recognition memory, working memory, and visual-motor response speed. This could be a great way of improving cognitive function amongst the elderly, anxiety and dementia.

HOW TO TAKE CINNAMON TO IMPROVE COGNITION

The simplest method to reap this benefit is to mix a few drops of cinnamon oil with a bit of carrier oil and diffuse the oil. For a bit of a boost, you can add about five drops of vanilla essential oil and two drops of orange essential oils. Diffuse this mixture.

MARY CONRAD

Chapter 11

Cinnamon as an Antioxidant

Antioxidants are chemicals that inhibit the oxidation of harmful chemicals, such as free radicals. The chemical processes in the body, which includes the metabolism, can lead to the production of free radicals. These free radicals can attach or bind to other molecules, leading to eventual build up and damage. An example of oxidation is when iron rusts when exposed to the environment. This is a similar process that could happen to your body when free radicals are not excreted.

HOW CINNAMON ACTS AS AN ANTIOXIDANT

Cinnamon has high levels of polyphenols. Phenolic compounds act as an antioxidant by "rapid donation" of hydrogen atoms and electrons to free radicals and lipids. These donations stabilize the radicals and significantly slows down the rate of propagation of the anti-oxidant chain since the molecule has become bulky. Polyphenols also trigger the production of glutathione, which is an essential component in detoxification.

A study used rats to gain insight on the antioxidant activity of cinnamon.

These rats were fed high fat diets then given either cinnamon or cardamom. The result was an increase in the antioxidant enzyme activities, which increased the glutathione levels. This countered the effects of the high fat intake.

The effects of cinnamon extract as an antioxidant is highly dependent on the extraction process, but it still proves to be a great source if natural antioxidants. Further human studies, need to be conducted to fully understand the use cinnamon for this benefit.

HOW TO USE CINNAMON AS AN ANTIOXIDANT

Adding cinnamon to your diet, is the simplest and most direct way of getting the antioxidant properties of cinnamon. Alternating it with turmeric, will give you the same effect with a different taste. Try cinnamon tea to start the day, and sprinkle some turmeric with a pinch of black pepper to your salad during lunch. It will definitely go a long way in improving your health with long term use.

PRECAUTIONS

Although amounts of less than 6 g, is considered safe, avoid intake if pregnant and nursing. Keep you stash of cinnamon away from children, as high amounts of cinnamon can cause itchiness and a burning sensation. This is especially true for those who have allergies to cinnamon.

Common signs of cinnamon allergy include:

- Runny nose
- Watery, itchy eyes
- Rashes after consuming cinnamon
- Upset stomach
- Swelling in the lips, throat or tongue
- Insomnia
- Shortness of breath

For any signs of excessive swelling and difficulty in breathing, emergency medical attention must be provided.

Chapter 12

Cinnamon as an Antifungal Agent

Antifungal agents refer to plants or pharmaceutical medications that inhibit the growth of fungi or have fungicidal properties. There are a lot of strains of fungus, including those that cause yeast infection.

An interesting fact is that cinnamon can also help with fungal infections in the nails, especially those in the toes. Toe nail fungus is one of the hardest to get rid of. This is commonly due to trauma when the nail bed separates from the nail and dies. The fungus begins to breed under the nail from moisture and creating a yellowish tinge on the surface.

The most common fungus responsible is dermatophyte fungus. The toe nail is more susceptible to fungus due to poor blood circulation and conducive environment for growth. Wearing socks that don't absorb moisture well or closed shoes, often raise the risks.

HOW CINNAMON ACTS AS AN ANTIFUNGAL AGENT

A study sought to determine the inhibitory effects of cinnamon on dermatophyte fungus. Since cinnamon had shown great antifungal properties on Candida species, they wanted to see if it also applies to other species of fungi.

The results indicated that the components of cinnamon, specifically cinnamaldehyde, eugenol and 0-methoxycinnamaldehyde, were mostly responsible for inhibiting fungal growth. Cinnamyl alcohol also exhibited antifungal properties in four strains of dermatophyte fungi. It works by increasing the permeability of the cell membrane, allowing the nutrients to leak out of the cell, which eventually leads to cell death.

HOW TO USE CINNAMON AS AN ANTIFUNGAL

Using cinnamon leaf oil, you can dilute it with a carrier oil and apply one drop to the affected area. A stronger effect can be obtained by applying 1 drop of 100% cinnamon leaf oil twice daily on the toe. Make sure to not put on too much, since it may cause irritation. For the first application, it would be best to dilute the oil to determine any possible allergic reaction.

A warm foot soak with Apple Cider Vinegar, and a pinch of Epsom salt would also help in drying the nail and getting rid of the fungus. Dilute cinnamon oil with a carrier oil, and massage the affected toe and feet to increase circulation. This will help increase antibodies in the affected area, which might help in fighting off the infection naturally.

PRECAUTIONS

Cinnamon oil can cause skin irritation, so always use small amounts to check if it's tolerated.

Toe nail fungus takes weeks to a year to cure. You can expect significant changes in about a week, but you also need to make sure that the oil seeps into the nail bed.

Chapter 13

Cinnamon for Alzheimer's disease

Alzheimer's disease is one of the leading causes of death among the elderly. Not all of these instances were a direct cause, but as an indirect result of the disease. This condition is marked by an irreversible and progressive decline in cognitive function. The person affected slowly loses his memory, reasoning and the ability to perform activities of daily living.

There is a loss of connection between neurons due to the clumping of amyloid plaques and neurofibrillary tangles. This causes the unpredictable behavior and changes in cognition.

SIGNS AND SYMPTOMS

There are early signs of Alzheimer's disease that shouldn't be overlooked. According to the Alzheimer's Association, the ten early warning signs of the disease include the following:

- Loss of memory that interrupts the activities of daily living
- Difficulty in planning or solving problems

- Unable to complete daily tasks
- Disorientation with regards to time and place
- Difficulty in understanding spacial concepts and visual images
- Sudden problems with written and spoken words
- Inability to retrace events or memories
- Poor judgement
- Withdrawal from social interaction and activities
- Changes in mood and personality

COMMON CAUSES OF ALZHEIMER'S DISEASE

It is believed that the main causes of Alzheimer's disease are a mixture of factors such as genetics, lifestyle and environment. These take a toll on the brain, which leads to irreparable damage. It is not fully known what really triggers this disease on a genetic level. The effect of the condition leads to brain cell death and loss of neural connections.

When doctors examined the brains of those who had Alzheimer's disease, they found two similar characteristics on all of them:

Amyloid Plaques: This is a buildup of protein substances that accumulates in the brain. It sticks to neurons, blocking connections and causing build up and damage.

Amyloid-beta precursor proteins are generally harmless, but when chemical processes break it down, beta-amyloid proteins are produced. This substance clumps together and easily adheres to neurons. It is also insoluble, which makes it difficult for the body to excrete.

Neurofibrillary Tangles: These are insoluble fibers in the neurons that are part of the microtubules that carry nutrients to the brain cells. These tangles are normally straight fibers, which are made up of tau proteins. In people with Alzheimer's disease, these tangles are collapsed, which in turn deprives the brain cells of nutrients. This eventually results in brain cell death.

HOW CINNAMON ACTS AGAINST ALZHEIMER'S DISEASE

The treatment for Alzheimer's disease focuses on palliative care. There is no specific cure, and existing treatments still require more study. Looking into a more natural method of prevention, studies have been conducted in vivo and in vitro to observe the effects of water-based cinnamon extract on both beta-amyloid plaques and neurofibrillary tangles.

The form of extract used had been stripped off of lipids, leaving only the water soluble compounds of C. zeylanicum. A study found that this extract stopped clumping of tau proteins and filament formation. It was discovered to completely alter the abnormal tau filaments, which promotes breakdown of the molecules. It was also noted that the effects of the extract didn't interfere with the normal process of microtubular formation. There were two compounds that had the most inhibitory effect: A-linked proanthocyanidin trimer molecule and cinnamaldehyde. The proanthocyanidin was removed during the purification of the extract but the cinnamaldehyde was retained.

In another study, a similar form of cinnamon extract was utilized to observe its effect on the formation of beta-amyloid plaques. The findings concluded that the extract was effective in stopping the formation of the plaques by interfering with the pathways necessary for the toxins to form. It was also noted that there was a recovery in cognitive function in the rats that were tested.

This can be seen as a potential prophylactic approach for Alzheimer's disease, as well as improving the quality of life for those who have the condition. As a natural remedy, this shows great potential in terms of halting the progression, but further studies is still needed.

HOW TO TAKE CINNAMON FOR PREVENTION

The safest way of taking cinnamon for this benefit is by adding it to your diet. Drinking cinnamon tea is a great way of slowly building the beneficial effects without having to worry about too many side effect. It can be adjusted as per your tolerated amounts, as long as it doesn't exceed the maximum recommended dosage.

Water-based based cinnamon extracts can also be taken in supplemental dosages. This is a more concentrated form of cinnamon where the harmful compounds in the lipids are stripped, leaving only the water-soluble molecules. This remedy still needs further study on its tolerance and dosages for human consumption.

PRECAUTIONS

Pregnant and nursing mothers, as well as children, should avoid taking oral supplemental dosages of cinnamon extract. Those with pre-existing conditions and are taking maintenance medications should consult with a physician before taking herbal supplements. Avoid taking cinnamon in conjunction with other herbs that have a similar effect, such as fenugreek, bitter melon, chromium, garlic or Panax ginseng. These herbs may interact with each other and lead to severe hypoglycemia.

Chapter 14

Cinnamon for Premenstrual Syndrome (PMS)

Premenstrual Syndrome is a set of symptoms experienced by women prior to menstruation. It might come as a surprise to women, but the symptoms must be severe enough to disrupt normal activities for it to be considered as PMS.

WHAT ARE THE CAUSES OF PMS?

The exact causes of PMS is not known, but it's attributed to the fluctuations of estrogen and progesterone that occurs prior to the onset of periods. Low levels of vitamins and minerals could also play a role in the severity of the symptoms. High sodium diet can also increase chances of PMS.

WHAT ARE THE SYMPTOMS OF PMS?

These are the common discomforts that women experience. It doesn't happen all at the same time, but may vary on the individual. Some months may have different set of symptoms than others:

- Slight weight gain
- Feelings of anxiety, irritability and depression
- Mood swings
- Increased appetite and food cravings
- Lower back pain
- Difficulty concentrating
- Fatigue
- Feeling bloated
- Breast tenderness
- Aggression

Dysmenorrhea is pain experienced before or during menstrual periods. It can range from mild discomfort to severe pain. It is caused by an increase in the production and release of prostaglandins during menstruation. The prostaglandins cause uterine smooth muscle contractions and gastrointestinal discomfort. It can result to nausea, vomiting and diarrhea.

HOW CINNAMON AFFECTS PMS

Cinnamon has been used traditionally to treat menstrual cramps. There are only a few studies which prove the efficacy of cinnamon in terms of managing pain from dysmenorrhea and reducing the symptoms of PMS.

According to the University of Maryland, low levels of manganese in the body may increase the intensity of PMS. Cinnamon is a rich source of manganese and calcium. Once these are addressed, the symptoms would be more tolerable.

A study conducted sought to find the effectiveness of cinnamon in relieving dysmenorrhea. It compared its effects between a control group (those who were given placebo pills), cinnamon group and ibuprofen.

It is well-known that cinnamon may be used as an anti-spasmodic. This is mainly due to cinnamaldehyde. It can help in reducing the smooth muscle contractions around the uterus. Another active component of cinnamon is eugenol, this compound can prevent the production of prostaglandin and decrease inflammation.

Pain measures were taken for each group to collect the data. The results found cinnamon to be more effective than the placebo group, but not as effective as ibuprofen. As a natural, non-pharmaceutical approach to pain, cinnamon can be effective.

HOW TO TAKE CINNAMON FOR PMS

It is always best to use Ceylon cinnamon due to its low levels of Coumarin. In a vegetable capsule, you can divide 2.5 grams of cinnamon powder in three divided doses. This can be taken a day before menstrual periods. It takes about 8 hours to take effect, so you can adjust accordingly.

To prevent PMS, you can take cinnamon tea daily for five days with two days of rest. This will help in preparing the body for menstruation, and keeping the symptoms mild.

PRECAUTIONS

Be mindful of the sodium content in food. Checking the labels is a good start in avoiding aggravated PMS. A balanced diet with lots of vegetables, fruits and regular exercise has proven effective for this condition. Keep hydrated during periods. Back rubs and hot packs are also effective non-pharmaceutical remedies to alleviate pain.

Check with your physician prior to taking supplemental dosages, especially if you're taking other maintenance medication. Avoid cinnamon supplements when pregnant, nursing and children below six years old.

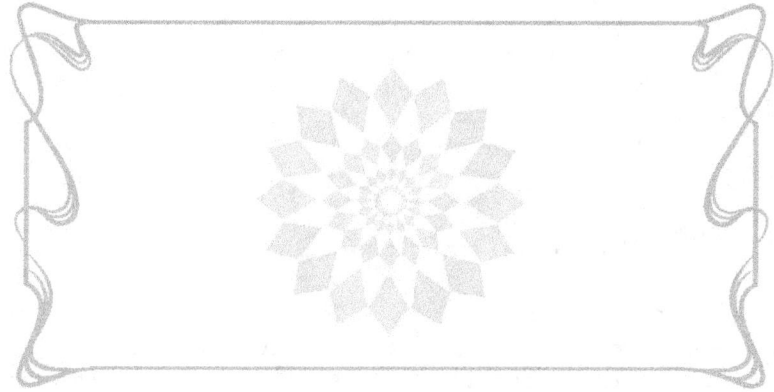

Chapter 15

Cinnamon for Stress Relief

Stress is a response to strain brought about unexpected events and demanding situations. In humans, stress activates our fight-or-flight response which is a survival instinct. This response is meant to ensure continuation of the species, but in today's context it can be for a number of reasons.

In stressful situations, the body responds by releasing corticosterone and norepinephrine. These hormones can spike up the heart rate, dilate the pupils, increase blood sugar levels, increases blood flow to the muscles, expands the bronchioles and decreases blood flow to the skin and intestines. This makes it optimal for the body to take action. In a life threatening situation, it can save you by enhancing your physical capabilities. In the workplace, it can temporarily boost your productivity. However, the stress response is actually self-limiting and wears off after a few hours.

The problem arises when stress becomes chronic. This happens when the perceived threat doesn't pass. A good example would be a demanding boss. In the beginning of the job, the stress placed upon your boss might boost your output but eventually it will decrease and crash. It can lead to health problems such as heart disease, anxiety and depression.

This makes it very important to manage stress by physical activities, a healthy diet, relaxation, massage and creating your own version of an orderly environment. Antioxidants can also reverse the effects of chronic stress in the body.

HOW CINNAMON AFFECTS STRESS

Stress hormones are produced by the adrenal glands. These hormones include corticosterone and norepinephrine. A recent study sought to determine how cinnamon affects stress levels through ulcer scoring, epinephrine and norepinephrine levels, blood glucose levels and cholesterol levels in the plasma.

The subjects were placed under a stressful environment for 21 days. The stress levels were measured and a marked increase in all factors were noted. The subjects were then given a dose of cinnamon at 200 mg/kg of weight. The results proved the anti-stress effects of cinnamon.

The ulcer scoring dropped after cinnamon was given. The levels of corticosterone decreased, which in turn allowed the mobilization of lipids. This decreased the cholesterol levels in the plasma. Norepinephrine release was mitigated, which stopped the increase of blood glucose.

Other than lowering the stress levels by affecting the adrenal glands, the scent of cinnamon can help with relieving stress and promoting relaxation.

HOW TO TAKE CINNAMON FOR STRESS RELIEF

Mix cinnamon oil with a carrier oil and diffuse it. It would infuse the environment with a mild scent. You can mix it with other essential oils that you favor.

Drink cinnamon tea to help you relax when anxious. For a more potent effect you can consult your herbalist or naturopathic doctor. This is for a safer and accurate dosage of cinnamon.

PRECAUTIONS

It's always best to avoid prolonged exposure to a stressful environment. If it can't be helped, frequent relaxation can go a long way in relieving stress. Find your best method of stress relief that is healthy, and keep practicing it.

If you're experiencing chest pains, shortness of breath and radiating pain, this could be a sign of a more serious problem. Please get checked out by a physician.

Chapter 16

Antiviral Properties of Cinnamon

A virus is a tiny infectious organism that spreads and grows by replicating within cells of other organisms. It can infect everything from plants, animal and even bacteria. Antivirals inhibit the replication process of viruses, but doesn't necessarily kill it.

HOW CINNAMON ACTS AS AN ANTIVIRAL

One of the earliest recorded use of cinnamon as an antiviral was published on March 1899 in the British Medical Journal. Dr. Charles Graham Grant discovered this particular property of cinnamon as he was in Ceylon (Sri Lanka). He had observed that people who were working in the cinnamon gardens were immune to the severe effects of malaria in the area. Upon this observation, he used cinnamon oil whenever he thought there was a need for an "internal antiseptic". In 1891, he endorsed the treatment to his fellow doctor, Dr. H.A. Stonham, who was encountering an influenza epidemic in his area. Both doctors were amazed at the positive results of the treatment. Dr. Grant then requested that cinnamon oil be considered as a general treatment.

It is best to note that this was studied with human patients, and even though it wasn't done with modern practices the results spoke volumes in terms of efficacy.

A more recent study also found that cinnamon had potential to control HIV infection and modulate immunity. They isolated a procyanidin polymer, IND02, and observed its effects on target cells. They had found that this polymer bonded to co-receptor binding site of infected cells. This inhibited interaction with the receptors of target cells which halted the spread of the virus. In addition, the presence of the polymer also enhanced the immune response to HIV.

Cinnzeylanine, which was extracted from C. zeylanicum, showed antiviral properties when examined under nuclear magnetic resonance analysis. It inhibited the spread of herpes simplex type 1 in Vero cells. Eugenol affects both type 1 and type 1 herpes simplex virus.

Other viruses that are inhibited by cinnamon include adenovirus (lung infections) and rotavirus (diarrhea).

HOW TO TAKE CINNAMON AS AN ANTIVIRAL

A safe way to get this benefit is by regularly taking cinnamon tea made with Ceylon cinnamon sticks. Adding cinnamon into your diet by sprinkling it on your salad, your banana smoothie or even in your coffee, would definitely make a difference!

For supplemental information, an herbalist would be able to provide effective and accurate information on how cinnamon can be taken to derive a more potent effect.

PRECAUTIONS

Further studies need to be done to determine a safe dosage when using cinnamon oil or cassia oil. These concentrated oils can irritate the mucosa and should only be taken internally with the advice of a health professional, herbalist or naturopathic physician. Cassia can also increase risks of liver problems due to its high levels of Coumarin.

Pregnant, nursing mothers and children should not take cinnamon oil.

Chapter 17

Cinnamon for ADHD

Attention Deficit Hyperactivity Disorder (ADHD) is a condition wherein there is an ongoing pattern of inattention or hyperactive behavior that interferes with normal development. This is a common condition among children but may extend to adulthood. It can result in poor performance in school, and trouble with learning.

The exact cause for ADHD is unknown, but there are several factors that play a role in its development.

- Genetics: Having family members who have ADHD increases the risk of developing this condition. Ongoing research is being conducted to determine which gene causes ADHD, but so far there has been no specific gene responsible for triggering it.

- Environment: Pregnant women who took drugs and alcohol increases the risk for their baby to eventually develop ADHD. There may be a need to modify a child's diet to eliminate sugar, food coloring and artificial flavors.

SIGNS AND SYMPTOMS OF ADHD

- Difficulty in paying attention
- Inability to stay still for short periods of time
- Impulsive behavior

HOW CINNAMON AFFECTS ADHD

Previous studies have confirmed that cinnamon has significant effects on cognitive function, Alzheimer's disease and in improving alertness. This study sought to determine the effects of cinnamon aromatherapy on children diagnosed with ADHD. The aromatherapy was done in conjunction with the usual rehabilitation treatments. This involved activity and cognitive training.

Twenty children were treated twice each week in 30-minute sessions. These children ranged from 2-7 years old. They were divided into two groups under experimental and control group. Both groups were placed in the same environment and same treatment course with only one variation. The experimental group received 1% cinnamon aromatherapy, which consisted of 1 gram of cinnamon in 100 ml of water. The control group were only given 100 ml of water. The progress was tracked for over half a year.

The results showed a significant improvement in the experimental group compared to the control group. Both groups actually improved under the rehabilitation treatment but the data indicated that there was a huge difference between both. This finding opens up the possibility of cinnamon aromatherapy as an alternative treatment for kids with ADHD.

HOW TO TAKE CINNAMON FOR ADHD

Diffusing cinnamon oil is the best way to yield its therapeutic effect. Prepare 1 drop of 100% cinnamon oil in 100 ml water during periods of activity to promote concentration and alertness.

PRECAUTIONS

Keep cinnamon oil away from places where children can reach. The oil is highly irritating to the mucosa and should not be ingested in concentrated doses.

Aromatherapy is an alternative treatment and may not be effective in all cases. It's a good alternative for a non-pharmaceutical approach to treating children.

MARY CONRAD

Conclusion

Thank you again for purchasing this book!

I hope this was able to help you learn about cinnamon and its benefits. It's truly fascinating to know that there is so much potential for the use of this spice to achieve health and wellness.

The next step is to visit an herbal store, grab good quality Ceylon cinnamon and consult with an herbalist and your doctor about the safety of using this spice.

Finally, if you enjoyed this book, then I'd like to ask you for a favor, would you be kind enough to leave a review for this book on Amazon? It'd be greatly appreciated!

Follow me on Twitter: @AuthorMConrad

Also, please like my Facebook page to get the latest news on my next book.

If you have any suggestions or specific natural remedies that you want to have researched and written, shoot me an email at authormaryconrad@gmail.com. I'm always on the lookout for great new topics to write about. :)

Have a great day!

Thank you and good luck!

MARY CONRAD

Author Biography

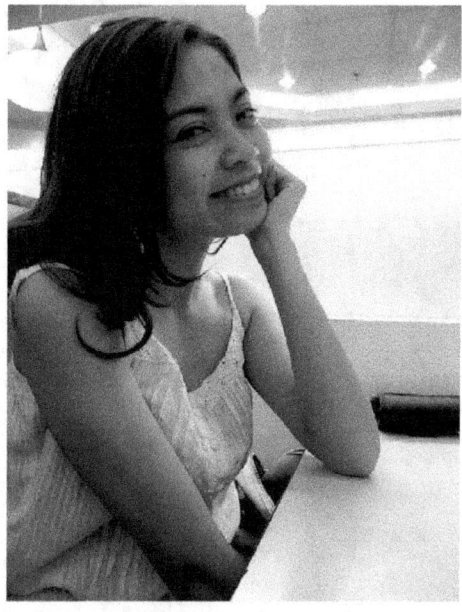

Mary Conrad is a Registered Nurse, who has a strong interest in natural remedies. As a mother, she believes in a holistic approach to health and well-being. Even though she graduated in the health profession, which usually advocates pharmaceutical medication, she believes that prevention is the best step towards health. Backed with scientific research, she wrote these books for both personal information and for others who share the same passion for holistic wellness. It's all about knowing the best natural ways to prevent disease and remedy current health problems. Like every health care provider, she believes in doing no harm, and promoting health. Take a step towards health, and towards nature.

References:

Chapter 1

Synan, M. (2013, October). Cinnamon's Spicy History. Retrieved February 08, 2016, from http://www.history.com/news/hungry-history/cinnamons-spicy-history

Cinnamon Health Benefits and Research. (n.d.). Retrieved February 11, 2016, from http://www.webmd.com/vitamins-and-supplements/lifestyle-guide-11/supplement-guide-cinnamon

Nutritional Profile: The Food Processor, Version 10.12.0, ESHA Research, Salem, Oregon, USA

Chapter 3

Kishore, P., MD. (n.d.). Diabetes Mellitus (DM) - Endocrine and Metabolic Disorders. Retrieved February 15, 2016, from http://www.merckmanuals.com/professional/endocrine-and-metabolic-disorders/diabetes-mellitus-and-disorders-of-carbohydrate-metabolism/diabetes-mellitus-dm

Gokhan S. Hotamisligil, M.D., Ph.D., professor of genetics and metabolism and chairman, Department of Genetics and Complex Diseases, Harvard School of Public Health, Boston; Christopher Newgard, Ph.D., director, Sarah W. Stedman Nutrition and Metabolism Center, and the W. David and Sarah W. Stedman Distinguished Professor, departments of pharmacology and cancer biology, biochemistry and medicine, Duke University Medical Center, Durham, N.C.; Oct. 15, 2004, Science

http://www.cinnamonvogue.com/cinnamon_for_diabetes.html

Chapter 4

Yeast Infections: MedlinePlus. (n.d.). Retrieved March 21, 2016, from https://www.nlm.nih.gov/medlineplus/yeastinfections.html

Yeast infection (vaginal). (n.d.). Retrieved March 21, 2016, from http://www.mayoclinic.org/diseases-conditions/yeast-infection/basics/definition/CON-20035129

Warnke, P. H., Becker, S. T., Podschun, R., Sivananthan, S., Springer, I. N.,

Russo, P. A., ... & Sherry, E. (2009). The battle against multi-resistant strains: renaissance of antimicrobial essential oils as a promising force to fight hospital-acquired infections. Journal of Cranio-Maxillofacial Surgery,37(7), 392-397.

Pires, R. H., Montanari, L. B., Martins, C. H. G., Zaia, J. E., Almeida, A. M. F., Matsumoto, M. T., & Mendes-Giannini, M. J. S. (2011). Anticandidal efficacy of cinnamon oil against planktonic and biofilm cultures of Candida parapsilosis and Candida orthopsilosis. Mycopathologia, 172(6), 453-464.

Chapter 5

Wang, L., Liu, F., Jiang, Y., Chai, Z., Li, P., Cheng, Y., ... & Leng, X. (2011). Synergistic antimicrobial activities of natural essential oils with chitosan films. Journal of agricultural and food chemistry, 59(23), 12411-12419.

Raybaudi-Massilia, R. M., Mosqueda-Melgar, J., & Martin-Belloso, O. (2006). Antimicrobial activity of essential oils on Salmonella enteritidis, Escherichia coli, and Listeria innocua in fruit juices. Journal of Food Protection®, 69(7), 1579-1586.

Friedman, M., Henika, P. R., & Mandrell, R. E. (2002). Bactericidal activities of plant essential oils and some of their isolated constituents against Campylobacter jejuni, Escherichia coli, Listeria monocytogenes, and Salmonella enterica. Journal of Food Protection®, 65(10), 1545-1560.

Chapter 6

Esmaillzadeh, A., Keshteli, A. H., Hajishafiee, M., Feizi, A., Feinle-Bisset, C., & Adibi, P. (2013). Consumption of spicy foods and the prevalence of irritable bowel syndrome. World J Gastroenterol, 19(38), 6465-6471.

Hawrelak, J. A., & Myers, S. P. (2010). Effects of two natural medicine formulations on irritable bowel syndrome symptoms: a pilot study. The Journal of Alternative and Complementary Medicine, 16(10), 1065-1071.

Chapter 7

Lee, C. W., Hong, D. H., Han, S. B., Park, S. H., Kim, H. K., Kwon, B. M., & Kim, H. M. (1999). Inhibition of human tumor growth by 2'-hydroxy-and 2'-benzoyloxycinnamaldehydes. Planta medica, 65(3), 263-266.

Ka, H., Park, H. J., Jung, H. J., Choi, J. W., Cho, K. S., Ha, J., & Lee, K. T. (2003). Cinnamaldehyde induces apoptosis by ROS-mediated mitochondrial permeability transition in human promyelocytic leukemia HL-60 cells.Cancer letters, 196(2), 143-152.

Koh, W. S., Yoon, S. Y., Kwon, B. M., Jeong, T. C., Nam, K. S., & Han, M. Y. (1998). Cinnamaldehyde inhibits lymphocyte proliferation and modulates T-cell differentiation. International journal of immunopharmacology, 20(11), 643-660.

Chapter 8

Tsuji-Naito, K. (2008). Aldehydic components of cinnamon bark extract suppresses RANKL-induced osteoclastogenesis through NFATc1 downregulation. Bioorganic & medicinal chemistry, 16(20), 9176-9183.

Tung, Y. T., Chua, M. T., Wang, S. Y., & Chang, S. T. (2008). Anti-inflammation activities of essential oil and its constituents from indigenous cinnamon (Cinnamomum osmophloeum) twigs. Bioresource Technology,99(9), 3908-3913.

Chapter 9

Prabuseenivasan, S., Jayakumar, M., & Ignacimuthu, S. (2006). In vitro antibacterial activity of some plant essential oils. BMC complementary and alternative medicine, 6

Deans, S. G., & Ritchie, G. (1987). Antibacterial properties of plant essential oils. International journal of food microbiology, 5(2), 165-180.

Singh, G., Maurya, S., & Catalan, C. A. (2007). A comparison of chemical, antioxidant and antimicrobial studies of cinnamon leaf and bark volatile oils, oleoresins and their constituents. Food and chemical toxicology, 45(9), 1650-1661.

Chapter 10

Cognitive Problem Symptoms, Causes and Effects. (n.d.). Retrieved March 21, 2016, from http://www.psychguides.com/guides/cognitive-problem-symptoms-causes-and-effects/

Zoladz, P. R., & Raudenbush, B. (2005). Cognitive enhancement through stimulation of the chemical senses. North American Journal of Psychology,7(1), 125-140.

Chapter 11

Su, L., Yin, J. J., Charles, D., Zhou, K., Moore, J., & Yu, L. L. (2007). Total phenolic contents, chelating capacities, and radical-scavenging properties of black peppercorn, nutmeg, rosehip, cinnamon and oregano leaf. Food chemistry, 100(3),

990-997.

Dhuley, J. N. (1999). Anti-oxidant effects of cinnamon (Cinnamomum verum) bark and greater cardamom (Amomum subulatum) seeds in rats fed high fat diet. Indian journal of experimental biology, 37, 238-242.

Muchuweti, M., Kativu, E., Mupure, C. H., Chidewe, C., Ndhlala, A. R., & Benhura, M. A. N. (2007). Phenolic composition and antioxidant properties of some spices. American Journal of Food Technology, 2(5), 414-420.

Chapter 12

Wang, S. Y., Chen, P. F., & Chang, S. T. (2005). Antifungal activities of essential oils and their constituents from indigenous cinnamon (Cinnamomum osmophloeum) leaves against wood decay fungi. Bioresource technology, 96(7), 813-818.

El Kady, & IA [القاضي الرزاق عبد اسماعيل]. (1993). Antibacterial and antidermatophyte activities of some essential oils from spices.

TOENAIL FUNGUS TREATMENT - NATURAL HOME REMEDY. (n.d.). Retrieved March 09, 2016, from http://www.cinnamonvogue.com/toenail_fungus_treatment_natural_home_reme dy.html

Chapter 13

Brion, J. P. (1998). Neurofibrillary tangles and Alzheimer's disease. European neurology, 40(3), 130-140.

Peterson, D. W., George, R. C., Scaramozzino, F., LaPointe, N. E., Anderson, R. A., Graves, D. J., & Lew, J. (2009). Cinnamon extract inhibits tau aggregation associated with Alzheimer's disease in vitro. Journal of Alzheimer's Disease, 17(3), 585-597.

Frydman-Marom A, Levin A, Farfara D, Benromano T, Scherzer-Attali R, Peled S, et al. (2011) Orally Administrated Cinnamon Extract Reduces β-Amyloid Oligomerization and Corrects Cognitive Impairment in Alzheimer's Disease Animal Models. PLoS ONE 6(1): e16564. doi:10.1371/journal.pone.0016564

Chapter 14

Manganese. (n.d.). Retrieved March 21, 2016, from http://umm.edu/health/medical/altmed/supplement/manganese

Jaafarpour, M., Hatefi, M., Khani, A., & Khajavikhan, J. Comparative Effect of Cinnamon and Ibuprofen for Treatment of Primary Dysmenorrhea: A Randomized Double-Blind Clinical Trial QC04-QC07.

Chapter 15

Saxena, B., & Saxena, U. (2012). Anti-stress effects of cinnamon (Cassia zelynicum) bark extract in cold restraint stress rat model. Int. J. Res. Dev. Pharm. L. Sci, 1(1), 28-31.

Chapter 16

Grant, CG. Correspondence: cinnamon in influenza. BMJ. 1899; 1: 763

Biedma, M. E., Connell, B., Schmidt, S., Lortat-Jacob, H., Moog, C., & Prakash, E. (2012). Anti-HIV and immune modulating activities of IND02.Retrovirology, 9(Suppl 2), P220.

Premanathan, M., Rajendran, S., Ramanathan, T., & Kathiresan, K. (2000). A survey of some Indian medicinal plants for anti-human immunodeficiency virus (HIV) activity. Indian Journal of Medical Research, 112, 73.

Benencia, F., & Courreges, M. C. (2000). In vitro and in vivo activity of eugenol on human herpesvirus. Phytotherapy Research, 14(7), 495-500.

Orihara, Y., Hamamoto, H., Kasuga, H., Shimada, T., Kawaguchi, Y., & Sekimizu, K. (2008). A silkworm–baculovirus model for assessing the therapeutic effects of antiviral compounds: characterization and application to the isolation of antivirals from traditional medicines. Journal of general virology, 89(1), 188-194.

Chapter 17

Attention Deficit Hyperactivity Disorder. (n.d.). Retrieved March 23, 2016, from http://www.nimh.nih.gov/health/topics/attention-deficit-hyperactivity-disorder-adhd/index.shtml

Symptoms of ADHD in Children, Teenagers, and Adults. (n.d.). Retrieved March 23, 2016, from http://www.webmd.com/add-adhd/tc/attention-deficit-hyperactivity-disorder-adhd-symptoms

Hui-Ming Chen, Hui-Wen Chen. THE EFFECT OF APPLYING CINNAMON AROMATHERAPY FOR CHILDREN WITH ATTENTION DEFICIT HYPERACTIVITY DISORDER. J Chin Med 19(1,2): 27-34, 2008 27

www.ingramcontent.com/pod-product-compliance
Lightning Source LLC
Chambersburg PA
CBHW071217280526
45787CB00002B/709